Amanda Baracho Trindade

Sex ratio of bovine embryos produced in vitro

Amanda Baracho Trindade

Sex ratio of bovine embryos produced in vitro

Literature review

ScienciaScripts

Imprint

Any brand names and product names mentioned in this book are subject to trademark, brand or patent protection and are trademarks or registered trademarks of their respective holders. The use of brand names, product names, common names, trade names, product descriptions etc. even without a particular marking in this work is in no way to be construed to mean that such names may be regarded as unrestricted in respect of trademark and brand protection legislation and could thus be used by anyone.

Cover image: www.ingimage.com

This book is a translation from the original published under ISBN 978-3-330-76819-2.

Publisher:
Sciencia Scripts
is a trademark of
Dodo Books Indian Ocean Ltd. and OmniScriptum S.R.L publishing group

120 High Road, East Finchley, London, N2 9ED, United Kingdom
Str. Armeneasca 28/1, office 1, Chisinau MD-2012, Republic of Moldova, Europe
Managing Directors: Ieva Konstantinova, Victoria Ursu
info@omniscriptum.com

Printed at: see last page
ISBN: 978-620-8-58362-0

SUMMARY

ACKNOWLEDGMENTS

To my parents for their unconditional encouragement, dedication, participation in my life and decisions, for never sparing any effort to provide me with a good quality education and, above all, for the example of life that I see in you.

To my brothers for their constant support, teachings and above all for their love and friendship.

To Alstyn for his understanding, companionship, support at all times when I needed it and for his patience in helping me make decisions.

To Professor Iveraldo Dutra for his guidance, collaboration, not only for adding technical knowledge, but mainly for teaching me how to handle each situation ethically, which was essential for my professional and personal development.

To Professor Alicio Martins Junior for the awakening that his classes gave me, for the technical training, which enabled me to do better in my curricular internship, and for his constant encouragement.

I would like to thank Professor Marcos Franke Pinto for giving me a deeper understanding of science by carrying out my first research project.

To Camila Frade for her trust and the opportunity to work as an intern, making it possible for me to have my first contact with the "world of IVF", for her teachings and encouragement, for her example of perseverance and discipline in a friendly and caring way.

To the team at Ativa Embriôes for welcoming me with open arms, for the trust placed in me, and especially for their willingness to contribute to my training, showing me that with ethics, honesty and respect new professionals can successfully enter the job market.

To the researcher Luiz Sergio de Almeida Camargo, for making my internship at Embrapa possible, which was essential for my professional growth and to the whole team at the animal reproduction laboratory, to Dudu, Michele Cristiny, Joâo Vitor, Myro, Carol, Bruno, Lilian, Michele Pereira, Fernanda Bernandes, Eliza, and especially to Joel, Samara, Fernanda Gonçalves, Bridgit, Alline and Josi for their affection and friendship.

To my friends from university, Tia, Bia, Isa, Bel, Borrega, Xuxu and Rodrigo, who shared incredible moments of my life with me over the last five years and who I'm sure will share many more,

To all those who, directly or indirectly, contributed to the completion of yet another stage.

INTERNSHIP REPORT

INTRODUCTION

The curricular internship was carried out in two places: Ativa Embryôes, for one month, and Empresa Brasileira de Pesquisa Agropecuâria (Embrapa), for three months, both in the city of Juiz de Fora - MG. The internship sites were chosen with the aim of improving and practicing the knowledge acquired during the degree.

Ativa Embrioes is a commercial *in* vitro fertilization (IVF) laboratory, a Vitrogen franchise, which is strategically located to serve producers in the Zona da Mata Mineira, Vertentes and the state of Rio de Janeiro. The company is made up of three partners: a veterinarian, a biologist and an administrator. The veterinarian provides assistance to dairy farms in the region, carrying out medical/surgical, reproduction and production services. The biologist carries out laboratory services and is the technical manager of the *in vitro* production (IVP) laboratory for bovine embryos. The other partner is responsible for the company's administration. The laboratory also has two other employees, another biologist who assists the technical manager and a secretary who, in addition to the duties expected of the position, also performs accounting services. Ativa Embriôes offers *ovum pick up* (OPU) services, IVP of bovine embryos, embryo transfer, pregnancy diagnosis, fetal sexing and embryo cryopreservation using the vitrification technique. As a result of partnerships with other companies, it offers DNA cell storage, cloning and DNA analysis services.

Embrapa's Animal Reproduction Laboratory (LRA) follows two main lines of research: Reproduction Biotechnology and Reproduction Physiology. The projects related to biotechnology carry out research into *in vivo* (ET) and *in vitro* embryo production, nuclear transfer (cloning) and transgenics. The other line of research includes studies of ovarian physiology, exogenous manipulation of reproductive function in dairy breeds, sexual behavior, reproductive management, the nutrient/reproduction relationship and thermal stress/reproduction. The experiments monitored by the intern were related to Reproductive Biotechnology, under the supervision of researcher Dr. Luiz Sergio de Almeida Camargo.

ACTIVE EMBRYONS

The laboratory is a Vitrogen franchise, so its procedures are standardized and established by that company, as are the means used.

Ativa Embrioes has a reception, an office and a laboratory, divided into three rooms. The first room is responsible for cleaning and sterilizing the materials. There is an autoclave, a drying and sterilizing oven, reverse osmosis water equipment, an ultrasonic washer, two sinks for washing hands and materials, a cupboard for storing materials and a sealing machine, a water bath and containers for storing semen. The second room contains a refrigerator and a freezer for storing media, aliquots and stock solutions, cabinets for storing materials in general and a precision scale. The last room is responsible for the production of embryos and can be accessed by passing through the other rooms. There are two desks, two incubators, a microcentrifuge, a microscope and a laminar flow where the embryo production procedures are carried out. In this flow there is a stereoscope, a heating plate, micropipettes and tips.

PROCEDURES FOR ENTERING THE LABORATORY

To enter the laboratory, it was compulsory to wear shoes, a lab coat and a cap. In the first room, hands were washed and dried with disposable paper towels. After these procedures, the hands were sanitized with 70% alcohol and so access could be gained to the embryo IVP room.

Activities monitored by the trainee

1. *IN VITRO* MATURATION (MIV)

1.1 Preparing the cryotubes

The day before the OPU, the 1.5 ml cryotubes were prepared with the washing medium. This was previously prepared at the beginning of the week, as it has a shelf life of seven days at refrigeration temperature. After being sealed with parafilm, the cryotubes were refrigerated and sent in a cooler box to the aspiration site. After OPU, the cryotubes were sent to the laboratory in an oocyte carrier, which kept them at 36°C.

1.2 Oocyte washing

The oocytes were removed from the cryotube along with the transport medium and placed in a Petri dish. In this plate, the oocytes were traced, transferred to a second plate, where they were washed twice in the washing medium and once in the maturation medium. After these procedures, the viable oocytes were counted and transferred to the maturation plate. Oocyte viability was analyzed by observing the cytoplasm, the number of cells making up the *cumulus* and their compactness.

1.3 MiV

The maturation plate was prepared the day before the OPU, containing the drops with maturation medium and coated with mineral oil, duly identified and kept in the incubator to stabilize. Oocytes from a donor were placed in each drop.

Incubation is carried out in a greenhouse at 38.8°C with an atmosphere of 5% carbon dioxide in atmospheric O2 and saturated humidity for 24 hours.

2. *IN VITRO* FERTILIZATION (IVF)

2.1 Mating

The mating was chosen by the farm owner together with the veterinarian in charge, according to the interests of each property. Most of the time, the semen was obtained from the centers and sent to the laboratory on the day of the OPU, being kept in a duly identified liquid nitrogen tank in a rack until it was used.

2.2 Sperm selection

To carry out IVF, the first step is sperm selection, carried out using a discontinuous Percoll gradient. This was always prepared minutes before fertilization began so that it could be heated in the incubation oven during this period. The dose of semen to be used was thawed in a water bath at 35°C and then the semen was placed in an eppendorf for subsequent transfer into the Percoll gradient (eppendorf). After this period, centrifugation was carried out, leaving only the *pellet* in the eppendorf, which was used for IVF.

2.3 Oocyte preparation

The IVF plates were prepared with the same number of drops as the maturation plates and were coated with mineral oil. These plates always remained in the incubator before the matured oocytes were transferred for stabilization. After 24 hours of maturation, the oocytes were washed twice, in a drop containing IVF medium, for subsequent transfer to the previously prepared IVF plate, following the same order as the maturation plate, in terms of donor identification.

2.4 IVF

After transferring the oocytes to the IVF plate, a pre-determined fixed amount of *pellet* from the Percoll was added to the drop containing the oocytes. The same incubation conditions imposed during maturation were maintained during this stage, which lasts 18 - 24 hours.

3. *IN VITRO* CULTIVATION (CIV)

3.1 Stripping

After approximately 22 hours of incubation of the sperm and oocytes, the IVF plate containing the probable zygotes was removed from the oven for denudation. After denudation, the probable zygotes were washed in IVC medium and then transferred to the IVC plate, following the same order as in the previous steps. Incubation was carried out under the same conditions as the other stages.

3.2 Feeding

On the third day of cultivation, the first feeding was carried out, which consisted of removing half the volume of medium from the drop and replenishing it with fresh CIV medium, previously stabilized in the incubator. On the same day, the cleaved structures were also counted, making it possible to calculate the cleavage rate of each drop. On the sixth day of development, another feeding was carried out, following the same procedures as the first.

3.3 Forecast

On the sixth day of development, along with feeding, an evaluation was carried out to check the blastocyst production rate. With this data, the veterinarian responsible for the transfer was notified, in order to program the management of the recipients the following day.

4. ENVASE

The embryos produced were transferred on the seventh day of development. The embryos from each animal were classified according to their stage of development and degree of embryonic quality, and then filled into 0.25 µL straws. The embryos were then transported to the transfer site in their own embryo carrier.

EMBRAPA

ACTIVITIES CARRIED OUT BY THE TRAINEE

1. *IN VITRO* EMBRYO PRODUCTION (PIV)

1.1 Follicular aspiration and oocyte retrieval

At the LRA, the ovaries used for oocyte retrieval came from slaughterhouse animals. After collection, the oocytes were placed in a thermos containing physiological solution (0.9% NaCl) at 37°C, plus streptomycin sulphate (50 mg/l) (solution 1), where they remained until they reached the LRA.

In the laboratory, the ovaries were washed twice in solution 1 and transferred to a beaker, where they remained in a water bath (36°C) until the follicles were aspirated. After these procedures, ovarian follicles between 2 and 8 mm in diameter were aspirated using a 10 ml syringe attached to a 25x8 mm needle. The follicular fluid containing the oocytes was slowly deposited on the wall of a conical glass cup kept in a water bath at 36°C.

Once the ovaries had been aspirated, the collecting cup containing the follicular fluid was kept in a water bath for 10-20 minutes, which was enough time for the oocytes to decant. The following steps were carried out in a laminar flow hood, without direct light, using a stereoscopic microscope and micropipettes.

Once the decantation was complete, the supernatant was discarded from the cell, leaving only the *pellet* with cells and oocytes. The next step was to trace the oocytes. To make this procedure easier, a Petri dish (100mm) with a checkered bottom was used. The traced oocytes were transferred to a second Petri dish containing washing medium (TALP HEPES) so that they could be classified according to the layer and compactness of the *cumulus* cells and the appearance of the cytoplasm.

1.2 *In vitro* maturation (IVM)

Oocytes with at least two layers of compact *cumulus* cells and homogeneous cytoplasm were selected and washed twice in TALP HEPES medium and once in maturation medium (TCM 199), in an excavated plate. The selected oocytes were then counted and transferred to the four-well maturation plate. This was prepared at least two hours before the start of maturation, so that each well contained 400 µL of TCM 199 for around 40-60 oocytes per well. Incubation took place in an incubator at 38.8°C with an atmosphere of 5% carbon dioxide, 20% oxygen and saturated humidity for 22 - 24 hours.

1.3 *In vitro* fertilization (IVF)

1.3.1 Sperm selection

In the LRA, sperm selection is carried out using the discontinuous Percoll gradient method (45% and 90%). The semen dose was thawed in a water bath at 37°C. After thawing, the semen was placed in an eppendorf containing the Percoll gradient. This was previously prepared and kept in the incubator to warm it up. The first centrifugation was carried out at 8000 RPM for seven minutes and the second at 3200 RPM for five minutes.

The semen was evaluated for vigor and motility after thawing and re-evaluated after thawing. Sperm concentration was measured using a Neubauer camera, 95 µL of distilled water and 5 µL of selected semen, making it possible to dilute the semen 20 times. Once the number of sperm has been obtained, it is possible to calculate the volume of semen needed to inoculate 2 x 106 per drop for fertilization.

1.3.2. Oocyte preparation

After 24 hours of maturation, the oocytes were washed twice in fertilization medium (FERT) and then transferred to the IVF plate. This had 70 µL drops of FERT medium coated with mineral oil, with 15-25 oocytes per drop indicated at this stage. The plate always remained in the incubator for at least four hours before the matured oocytes were transferred, to stabilize the medium and the oil.

1.3.3 IVF

After preparing the semen and transferring the oocytes to the IVF plate, the ideal volume of semen was transferred to obtain a concentration of 2×10^6 sperm per drop. This was topped up with FERT medium so that the final volume was 100 µL. The same incubation conditions were maintained for this stage, which lasts between 18 and 24 hours.

1.4 *In vitro* culture (IVC)

It occurs around 22 hours after fertilization begins, after which time the probable zygotes undergo total or partial denudation of the *cumulus* cells.

1.4.1 Stripping

Denuding can be mechanical or enzymatic, depending on the atmosphere of the incubator.

In mechanical stripping, the IVF drop is pipetted several times, causing the probable zygotes to come into contact with each other, which helps to mechanically remove the *cumulus* cells. The probable zygotes were then washed in CIV medium (CR2) and transferred to a plate with 50 µL drops of CR2, coated with mineral oil, where up to 15 structures per drop were indicated. Incubation was carried out under the same conditions as the previous stages.

When the probable zygotes were going to be cultivated in a controlled atmosphere with 5% oxygen and 90% nitrogen, denudation was carried out in order to remove all the cells around the probable zygote, for which enzymatic denudation was carried out. The probable zygotes were removed from the drop and placed in a Falcon tube (15 mL) containing 1mL of hyaluronidase. The tube was subjected to mechanical agitation for five minutes so that complete denudation could occur. After this period, the probable zygotes were transferred to a Petri dish and the Falcon tube was washed three times with TALP medium to recover the structures. These were traced in the Petri dish, washed once in CR2 medium for subsequent transfer to the culture plate, a four-well plate with 400 µL of CR2 and 90 µL of mineral oil.

1.4.2. Feeding

On the third day of cultivation, the first feeding was carried out, removing half (25 µL) of the drop medium and replenishing it with fresh CIV medium, previously stabilized in an oven at 38.8°C with a 5% carbon dioxide atmosphere. At the time of feeding, the cleaved structures were evaluated to obtain the cleavage rate.

In the oxygen-controlled greenhouse, there was no need for feeding due to the amount of medium per well (400 µL), so only the cleaved structures were counted.

On the seventh day of culture, the embryos were classified according to their stage of development and embryonic quality.

2. PRODUCTION OF TRANSGENIC EMBRYOS

Transgenics is a technique that aims to produce animals that have a stable incorporation of an exogenous DNA fragment, transferring these genes to their offspring (GONÇALVES *et al.,* 2008). Interest in the production of transgenic animals is related to the pharmaceutical industry, animal production and medicine.

Some biopharmaceuticals are in the final stages of testing and their production is aimed at the mammary gland of some species, such as: production of antithrombin III in goats, production of human serum albumin in cows, production of coagulation factor IX in sheep. With regard to animal production, genetic modification aims to increase weight gain, carcass quality, milk production, prolificacy, modify milk composition and produce animals resistant to diseases. Another advantage of transgenics is the use of xenotransplants, used as an alternative to meet the demand, since the ratio of donors to patients is 1:4 (RUMPF & MELO, 2005).

The incorporation of exogenous DNA can be carried out by various methods, the most common being the transfection of exogenous DNA by liposomes, by electroporation, transduction by viral vectors (BRESSAN, 2008), by pronuclear injection and nuclear transfer (RUMPF & MELO, 2005).

Retroviral vectors have RNA as their genetic material and, when they infect mammalian cells, they convert it into DNA, which is integrated into the host cell. However, the animals produced by this technique have a low rate of transmission of the transgene to their offspring (RUMPF & MELO, 2005). When the method of choice is liposome transfection, the DNA is introduced into the cells by fusing the lipid-DNA complex with the cell membranes. In electroporation, the DNA of interest is incubated in a solution with the target cells and this solution is subjected to electrical pulses that destabilize the membrane, causing pores that allow the DNA to enter (BRESSAN, 2008). Another method for introducing exogenous genes is pronuclear injection, which consists of the direct introduction of exogenous DNA into one of the pro-nuclei formed during the initial stage of oocyte fertilization, and is the most successful method for producing transgenic animals. With regard to nuclear transfer, transfection is carried out in nucleus donor cells, which are fused to the recipient cytoplasm (RUMPF & MELO, 2005).

One of the LRA's lines of research is the production of transgenic embryos using different techniques. In one of the lab's experiments, for example, transfection was carried out, using nanoparticles as vectors and a reporter gene to evaluate the technique.

3. GAUGING THE GAS ATMOSPHERE IN INCUBATORS

Its purpose is to control the CO2 level in the incubators, a procedure based on the operating manual for the equipment (Fyrite) used to measure gases (O2 and CO2) in incubators.

The LRA protocol for carrying out this procedure is:

- Check that the liquid inside the meter is at the zero mark before calibrating;
- Press the valve at the top of the meter 03 times to remove the air;
- Connect one end of the rubber cable to the oven and the other to the appliance;

- Fill the pump by pressing it 18 times;
- Pour the liquid twice into the meter;
- Check the CO_2 volume recorded;

The control was carried out weekly (every Monday) and the value found was noted on the form for each greenhouse, as well as the date and name of the person responsible for the procedure.

4. WASHING AND STERILIZING MATERIALS

All the materials used in the laboratory, with the exception of culture tips and plates, were reused and had to be properly washed and sterilized.

4.1 Cleaning glassware

All the glassware used was washed with soap and water, rinsed ten times in tap water and five times in distilled water, and then transferred to a solution of 10% nitric acid, where it remained for 45 minutes. After this period, the glassware was rinsed ten times in tap water and five times in distilled water, and then sterilized in an oven at 150°C for one hour and thirty minutes.

4.2 Cleaning and sterilization of plastics

Plastics, such as Falcon tubes, were washed after use and immersed in a 10% nitric acid solution for up to a week. After this period, they were washed ten times in tap water, five times in distilled water and placed in a drying oven (60°). Proper packaging was carried out using plastic bags and a sealing machine, so that the plastics were stored. Sterilization was carried out using the autoclaving process, which aims to eliminate all microorganisms.

The tips used were not packed in boxes but in their own packaging and sterilized in the same way as the other plastics.

4.4 Sterilization of bacteriological filters

The aim of this procedure is to clean the bacteriological filter holders that were used to filter the culture media, as they are not disposable. After use, the filter holders were washed ten times in tap water and five times in distilled water and then dried in an oven. Once dry, they were wrapped in brown paper and sterilized in an autoclave.

5. PREPARATION OF GROWING MEDIA

All the culture media were produced in the LRA itself by an employee, a veterinary doctor, trained to carry out this procedure. The stock media were made every fifteen days and remained under refrigeration (8°C) during this period. The "ready to use" media were made daily and remained in the incubator for at least two hours before use, for prior stabilization.

For maturation, the culture medium used at the LRA was TCM 199, the only non medium produced in the laboratory. According to Gonçalves *et al.* (2007), this is the most widespread medium among IVP laboratories and is usually supplemented with fetal bovine serum, FSH, LH, pyruvate and antibiotics, although there are variations between laboratories.

The culture medium used during the IVF stage was FERT TALP, which according to Gonçalves *et al.* (2007) contains factors capable of promoting sperm capacitation, such as heparin, and is the medium most commonly used in laboratories during *in vitro* fertilization.

The medium chosen by LRA for IVC is CR2, which has a longer shelf life than the others and can be used for seven days when stored under refrigeration.

6. COURSES

During my internship, I took two courses offered by Embrapa: Update in Dairy Cattle and TecLeite. The first course lasted 28 hours and covered various topics on dairy cattle, with the lectures on dairy cow reproduction and nutrition being the most important, as they are related to the area of choice for the internship. The second course lasted four hours and covered topics on reproductive biotechnology in cattle, which was an excellent complement to the internship.

The courses were important because, as well as gaining more information about the field, it was possible to make contact with experienced professionals and share information with other students.

7. CONCLUSION

Compulsory curricular internships are an important stage in academic training, where we put into practice the knowledge acquired during our degree, adding to our knowledge and experience, which makes a difference to our professional training.

The internship at Ativa Embriões allowed me to get to know the commercial routine, realizing the practical skills of the professional in charge, as well as the care and attention required to carry out any procedure. It was interesting to see how the selection of donors and bulls influences the genetic improvement of the herd, and how quickly this can happen with IVP of bovine embryos, which increased my vision of the process, providing great professional growth.

My internship in a research laboratory showed me that the technological advances and efficiency of commercial laboratories exist because of the intense study to improve techniques that takes place in research centers.

8. BIBLIOGRAPHICAL REFERENCES

BRESSAN, F.B.; **Production of transgenic animals by nuclear transfer as a biological study model.** 2008. 80p. Master's dissertation: Faculty of Veterinary Medicine and Zootechny. University of Sao Paulo. Pirassununga, 2008

RUMPF, R.; MELO, E.O.; Production of transgenic animals: methodology and applications. **Documentos/ Embrapa recursos genéticos e biotecnologia**, v. 145, p. 110- 145, 2005.

GONCALVES, P. B. D. ; BARRETA, M.H. ; SANDRI, L.R. ; et al. In vitro production of bovine embryos: the state of the art. **Revista Brasileira de Reproduçâo Animal,** v. 31, p. 212-217, 2007.

GONCALVES, P.B.D.; FIGUEIREDO, J.R.; FREITAS, V.J.F. **Biotechniques applied to animal reproduction**. Sao Paulo: Varela, 2008.

LITERATURE REVIEW

SUMMARY

Brazilian cattle farming plays an extremely important role in the food industry and needs to be increasingly efficient in order to meet market needs at a lower production cost. Reproductive biotechnologies are important tools that help to increase production rates, providing high gains in animal production. *In* this sense, *in vitro* embryo production stands out because it is the biotechnique that enables the highest number of offspring per female, which is reflected in rapid genetic gain, a reduction in the interval between generations and a rapid increase in the herd. However, there are several reports that this technique causes sexual disproportion of the embryos, with more male embryos being observed, which can be detrimental given the need for a certain gender, according to each production system. Knowledge of the factors involved in the process of disproportion between the sexes of bovine embryos produced *in vitro* will provide subsidies for improving the technique, for cattle breeding, for increasing rates and for reducing production costs. The aim of this review is to discuss the main factors involved in sex ratio deviation, as well as the importance of this for cattle breeding.

Keywords: sex, disproportion, embryo, male, *in vitro* fertilization

INTRODUCTION

1.1 Cattle farming in the world

The modern cattle industry is the result of a slow evolution of breeding techniques developed over decades, and is dependent on management, health, genetic improvement and reproduction programs (SEVERO, 2009). The main purpose of cattle farming worldwide is to produce quality, safe food for the population.

India has the largest beef herd in the world, leaving Brazil in second place in the ranking, which represents 18.6% of the world herd, according to the Minas Gerais State Secretariat for Agriculture, Livestock and Supply (2011). Also according to the Secretariat, Brazil is currently the world's largest beef exporter, contributing 20.7% of exports.

Milk production in our country has grown significantly in recent years, as 13.8% of the world's lactating cows are in Brazil, ranking it third internationally in terms of the largest herd of dairy cattle. However, we only contribute 6.9% of world production, ranking eighth among the largest producers. The United States, on the other hand, has 6.9% of lactating cows in relation to the world herd, but is in a more competitive position than us, because it ranks third in the world ranking of milk production, contributing 16.9% (Secretaria de Estado de Agricultura, Pecuària e Abastecimento de Minas Gerais, 2011).

This data, coupled with the growing demand for food, highlights the need to improve production efficiency. It is therefore essential to use new technologies to increase herd productivity and, as a result, enable Brazil to achieve more competitive positions in the international milk market and become even more qualified in the world beef market.

1.2 Cattle farming in Brazil

Brazilian cattle farming is of significant economic and social importance and stands out on the international stage for its growth potential and the size of its herd, estimated at

209,541,109 (IBGE, 2010). The region with the largest cattle herd in Brazil is the Midwest, with 34.6%, followed by the North with 20%, and in third place, the Southeast, representing 18.2% of the total national herd (IBEGE, 2010).

Meat production in 2012 is expected to reach 25.3 million tons. This figure is influenced by domestic consumption, exports and increased productivity. Bovine milk production reached 30.7 billion liters *in* 2010, and the volume of *fresh* milk exported that year was 8.802 tons (IBGE, 2011).

1.3 Reproductive biotechnology and cattle breeding

As cattle farming grows in Brazil, so does the need and importance of incorporating new technologies into the production sector. Neves *et al.* (2010) highlight the importance of technological progress in livestock farming and that, with this thesis, they have had a major academic impact with repercussions in the production sector, a fact that proves the viability of developing technological innovations. Furthermore, these techniques have been a decisive milestone in the development of world livestock farming and, as a result, have caused major economic development and a notable impact on income (THIBIER, 2005).

According to Thibier (2005), the first generation of biotechniques was artificial insemination (AI), followed by embryo transfer (ET), then *in vitro* fertilization (IVF) along with embryo sexing and animal cloning and, finally, the production of transgenic animals. Thus, it can be seen that the implementation of these biotechniques is the basis for genetic improvement programs, since these programs use these techniques to select individuals with characteristics that are desirable for production such as: greater weight development, carcass yield, milk production, better feed conversion and sexual precocity and thus make it possible to increase productivity (BARUSELLI *et at.*, 2006 ; PINEDA, 2004).

1.4 Artificial insemination

Artificial insemination was the first biotechnology used in animal reproduction. It was initially used in cattle, with the aim of genetic improvement through the use of semen from superior bulls with characteristics of interest (GONÇALVES *et al.,* 2008). In our country, in 2011, around 10% of the matrices in the national herd were inseminated through AI (ASBIA, 2011).

The technique has several advantages, such as genetic improvement through the use of semen from bulls with high genetic value, control of venereal diseases, an increase in the number of offspring per sire, and the transmission of the bull's genetic characteristics even after death through semen freezing (BEARDEN *et al.*¡2003). However, the success of artificial insemination depends on the detection of oestrus, which, according to Severo (2009), is responsible for the main failure in an AI program. Postpartum anestrus, late puberty and the limitation of obtaining only one calf per cow are also disadvantages of AI (BARUSELLI *et al.*, 2006).

1.5 Fixed-time artificial insemination

Fixed-time artificial insemination (FTAI) is an improvement on AI because, according to Bó *et al.* (2003), it can be used to reduce the problem of detecting oestrus. Other advantages of FTAI are that it avoids the problems of post-partum anestrus, concentrates the return of heat for breeding and optimizes manpower. This is because this technique makes it possible to inseminate a large number of cows in a short period of time, and consequently concentrates the birth of calves (BARUSELLI *et al.*, 2006).

Like any technique, IATF also has disadvantages, the main one being the response of each animal to hormone treatment, which can make the technique unfeasible. Therefore, the program depends on the cost/benefit ratio (BARUSELLI *et al.*, 2006).

1.6 Transfer of *in vivo* produced embryos

The second generation of biotechnology is *in vivo* embryo transfer (ET), a technique that has been used in livestock farming for over thirty years (THIBIER, 2005).

TE makes it possible to produce a greater number of offspring per female during her reproductive life, and is one of the most economical methods for increasing the reproductive rates of females with high genetic value (GONÇALVES *et al.,* 2008). However, this biotechnique also has its disadvantages, such as the lower number of embryos that can be produced and transferred per female and the hormonal treatment that must be carried out on them. These factors do not occur with *in vitro* embryo production (THIBIER, 2005), highlighting the main advantages of this biotechnique.

In 2005, it was found that more than 500,000 embryos produced *in vivo* are transferred worldwide, with Brazil being responsible for approximately ¼ of these transfers (THIBIER, 2005). However, from 2006 to 2011, there was a 73% decrease in the production of *in vivo* embryos in Brazil and a 28% increase in embryos produced *in vitro*, which can be explained by the need to speed up production, combined with the costs involved and the current rates of production using the *in vitro* technique (DIAS, 2012).

1.7 *In vitro* embryo production

In vitro embryo production (IVP) began in Europe in the 1990s, but expanded in Japan and Brazil (THIBIER, 2005). Our country is currently the largest producer of *in vitro* embryos, accounting for approximately 85% of world production (DIAS, 2012).

The technique has a number of advantages, including: collecting oocytes from cows that have died; recovering oocytes from females at stages that other techniques don't allow, including in the gestation; the greater quantity of oocytes collected per female compared to other biotechniques; independence from hormonal treatment; speeding up the production of genetically superior animals and helping other techniques. Another important advantage is that it prevents the early disposal of genetically privileged females with acquired alterations that prevent reproduction from occurring naturally (GONÇALVES *et al.*, 2008).

According to Thibier (2005), this biotechnology has great potential in the future compared to others and will probably be the most widely used in the world. This is due to the opening up of new international markets interested in buying genetics to improve their herds, the fact that animals with a high genetic content will stand out as providers of superior characteristics in food production, sustaining market demand (DIAS, 2012), as well as the healthiness of the technique, the help in preserving endangered species and the possibility of reducing costs (THIBIER, 2005).

1.8 Transgenics

Transgenics is a technique that aims to produce animals that have a stable incorporation of an exogenous DNA fragment, transferring these genes to their offspring (GONÇALVES *et al.,* 2008). According to this author, the use of this biotechnique will have a major impact on improving efficiency, since according to Neves *et al.* (2010) there is rapid multiplication of animals with desirable characteristics.

1.9 The importance of sex in cattle farming

Sex determination in cattle farming, both beef and dairy, can be one of the determining factors in improving the productive and economic performance of the activity. An example of this is male calves on dairy farms, which have little or no zootechnical value. On the other hand, on commercial beef farms, the male calf is the sex of interest due to its greater production potential.

It can be seen that a particular gender can favor the productivity of each specific system, according to its needs. It is therefore possible to see that gender selection has a significant economic value for animal production.

1.10 Objective

The aim of this review is to address the factors that influence the sex ratio of *in vitro* produced embryos and to report on the aspects of this technology for the better development of national livestock farming.

MATERIAL AND METHODS

The strategy for this literature review consisted of searching for scientific articles, books and theses on *in vitro* embryo production, sex determination, sex ratio and factors involved *in* this process.

We consulted the local collections of the libraries of the Universidade Estadual Paulista - Campus de Araçatuba and Embrapa Gado de Leite, as well as books on reproductive biotechniques. Scientific articles were searched on scientific publication sites such as Scielo, PubMed, Science Direct and Google Scholar.

The criterion for selecting books, articles and theses was the amount of relevant information provided. Books, articles and theses that offered vague or little information on the subject were disregarded.

LITERATURE REVIEW

1.11 Importance and justification of PIV

In artificial insemination, efforts are focused on increasing productivity by using breeding stock with proven genetic merit (SILVA *et al.*, 2007). The success of the technique depends on the detection of oestrus, which can be difficult in *Bos indicus* females, as they have a tendency to present oestrus during the night and with a shorter duration than *Bos taurus* (BÓ *et al.*, 2003). Social hierarchy can also play a influence on the identification of signs of oestrus, since dominant cows tend not to allow mounting, masking identification by this criterion (GALINA *et al.*, 1996).

With the development of IATF protocols, heat detection has become unnecessary, as both the day of insemination can be programmed and the calf birth season (BARUSELLI *et al.*, 2004), which consequently concentrates labor. However, it's important to note that in both AI and IATF, one calf is obtained per cow over the period of one year, while in the transfer of embryos produced *in vivo* and *in vitro*, this ratio is higher.

According to GALLI *et al.* (2003), *in vitro* embryo production was developed as a research tool and used to rescue oocytes from slaughterhouse animals. The follicular puncture technique (*ovum pick up* - OPU) is the most respected in the use of live donor oocytes for *in vitro* fertilization (IVF). Its advantage is that it doesn't interfere with the donor's normal productive cycle, as it means that hormone treatment, an essential procedure in ET, is no longer necessary.

According to Bols *et al.* (1997), in TE each embryo donor can multiply the number of offspring in her reproductive life by more than three times. In IVP, four times more embryos can be produced than in TE (KRUIP *et al.*, 1994), but at a higher cost per embryo (RODRIGUES & GARCIA, 2000; RUMPF, 2007). It is known that the female bovine has approximately 70,000 oocytes in her ovaries at the time of puberty (HAFEZ, 2000), generating approximately ten offspring throughout her reproductive life (BOLS *et al.*, 1997). With the use of OPU, each female bovine is capable of producing 50 to 100 embryos/year, through a regimen of two punctures per donor per week for several months (GONÇALVES *et al.*, 2008).

OPU makes it possible to retrieve oocytes from both pre-pubertal females (RUMPF, 2007; GALLI & LAZZARI, 1996; KRUIP *et al.*, 1994) and those with reproductive problems (GALLI, *et al.*, 2003; NEVES *et al.*, 2010; RUMPF, 2007, GARCIA *et* al., 2004; GONÇALVES *et al.*, 2007; GONÇALVES *et al.*, 2008), as well as pregnant or senile women (RUMPF, 2007; GONÇALVES et al., 2007; GONÇALVES *et al.*, 2008). This type of procedure makes it possible to reduce the interval between generations, without the need to remove these donors from the production system, which overcomes one of the drawbacks of TE, which is precisely the removal of elite cows from the production system (FERREIRA *et al.*, 2001). There is also a constant supply of F1 embryos for milk or meat production programs (RUMPF, 2007), which helps to increase productivity and profit in the activity.

Among the challenges of IVP is the high cost of the OPU procedure and the dedication required to train in the technique (SENEDA *et al.*, 2006). However, improvements in the OPU technique and *in vitro* culture conditions have made it possible to apply IVP on a commercial scale (GONÇALVES *et at.*, 2007), as well as the optimization of IVP, involving the production of good quality embryos in increasingly large numbers, associated with the reduction of the problems mentioned above, contribute to a decrease in its operating cost, making it possible to disseminate this technology with the aim of increasing the productivity of national livestock (GARCIA *et al.*, 2004). Although embryo cryopreservation is constantly being studied, it is still a limiting factor in IVP (RUMPF, 2007).

1.12 Practical implications of sexual difference for cattle farming

Since the 1970s, with the embryo transfer technique, the animal industry has aimed to determine the sex of embryos before transfer (THIBIER, 1995). In an attempt to select the sex of mammals, species of zootechnical interest, companion animals, endangered species and assisted human reproduction, a series of technologies are used (HOSSEPIAN DE LIMA, 2007).

In dairy farming, a practical example of the importance of sex is the creation of specialized breeds, because according to Hossepian de Lima (2007) the maintenance of pregnancies and the birth of male animals is one of the factors that reduce productivity and increase production costs. In these herds, sex selection would reduce or eliminate the cost of producing calves, as well as producing genetically superior replacement calves, by classifying cows and bulls according to the estimated genetic merit for milk production characteristics (LUCIO, 2007).

In beef cattle farming, the difference in carcass characteristics, as shown by Ruvuna *et al.* (1992), the dead weight of males at 24 months is around 25% higher than the dead weight of females of the same age.

Since gamete production is constant, the number of males with high zootechnical potential needed in a herd is much smaller than the number of females. The devaluation of male products can be explained by the fact mentioned above and by the low probability of a calf becoming a semen donor. As far as females are concerned, every heifer from a well-planned mating is potentially a future donor, thus justifying the higher value placed on female products (RUFINO, 2006).

1.13 Factors influencing sex ratio

1.13.1 *In vitro* cultivation conditions

In the *in vitro* embryo production system, a deviation in the male:female ratio has been observed, where the percentage of male embryos is higher than the theoretically expected 1:1. The factors that influence the sex ratio of embryos produced *in vitro* have been the subject of debate.

Several authors agree that the conditions imposed by the culture can influence embryo growth rates (AVERY *et al.*, 1989a; GUTIERREZ *et al.* 1996; GRISART *et al.,* 1995), as well as the medium and its components. These factors can alter the survival of female embryos and consequently affect the sex ratio (BREDBACKA & BREDBACKA, 1996 a ; GRISART *et al.* 1995; KOCHHAR *et al.* 2001).

Some authors (HOLM *et al.*, 1998; KOCHHAR *et al.*, 2003) report that the conditions of the embryo culture medium can interfere with the kinetics of development, thus altering the duration of cell cycles. According to Kochhar *et al.* (2003), in most species, embryos produced *in vitro* fall into two defined groups in the first few days of development: fast cleavage and slow cleavage, in which there is,

respectively, a predominance of males and females, with cleavage rates and speeds in the first days of culture favoring male embryos (BREDBACKA & BREDBACKA, 1996 b; AVERY *et al.*, 1989). During *in vitro* culture, male zygotes generally cleave first (BREDBACKA & BREDBACKA, 1996 a and b; DOMINKO & FIRST, 1997) and reach the blastocyst stage faster than females (AVERY *et al.* 1992; GUTIÉRREZ-ADAN *et al.*,1996; PEGORARO *et al.*, 1998).

Pegoraro *et al.* (1998) showed that male embryos develop faster than female embryos when cultured in *vero cells* and bovine oviduct cells (BOEC). Also in this experiment, the variation in the sex ratio was observed in both culture systems, being more pronounced in more advanced stages (expanded blastocysts).

Gutiérrez-Adân *et al.* (2001) showed that media containing synthetic oviduct fluid (SOF) influences the sex of blastocysts, since in that study male embryos were in greater proportion. However, Grisart *et al.* (1995) found no differences in sex ratio when blastocysts were produced in SOF medium.

According to Gutierréz-Adan *et al.* (1996), in the presence of fetal bovine serum (FBS), male embryos develop faster and with better quality than female embryos. In another experiment (GUTIERRÉZ-ADAN *et al.*, 2001), FBS again caused a shift in the ratio, favoring males until the sixth day of culture, and after the ninth day there was a balance in the ratio. However, Gilardi *et al.* (2004) observed no influence of SFB on the development of female or male embryos and the 1:1 ratio in embryos seven or eight days post-fertilization was maintained. In the same study, bovine serum albumin (BSA) also did not alter the sex ratio.

According to Merighe *et al.* (2010), the combination of *in vitro* culture conditions and an imbalance in the levels of metabolically important enzymes at the beginning of development can be detrimental to the development of female embryos. The difference in sex ratio may be related to the ability of male embryos to withstand stress during the early stages of development (AVERY *et al.*, 1989, 1992; GUTIÉRREZ-ADÂN *et al.*, 2001).

1.13.2 Glucose

Glucose, a molecule that occupies a central position in the production of energy and the synthesis of complex molecules (RIEGER, 1992), is one of the most important substrates for *in vitro* cultured embryos, but in high concentrations it can be harmful to bovine embryonic development (IWATA *et al.*, 1998).

It is known that male and female embryos have different metabolic requirements when cultured *in vitro*. In relation to glucose, this requirement is twice as high in male embryos as in females, and the activity of the pentose phosphate pathway (PPP) is four times better in female blastocysts than in males (TIFFIN *et al.*, 1991).

Several authors have observed that male bovine embryos, when cultured in a medium containing glucose, cleave more quickly than female embryos (BREDBACKA & BREDBACKA, 1996 b; PEIPPO *et al.*, 2001; KOCHHAR *et al.*, 2001; PEIPPO & BREDBACKA, 1996). Parrish *et al.* (1995) also support this idea, because when embryos were cultured in a high concentration of glucose, an increase was found in the proportion of males in relation to females. In the case of cultivation in the absence of glucose, there was a shift in the sex ratio, with a higher number of female embryos. When the concentration of glucose was reduced, the sex ratio remained unchanged at 50% of each sex.

Peippo *et al.* (2001) maintain the same position with regard to this idea, as they found that embryo sex is affected by the timing of cleavages in the presence or absence of glucose in the culture medium. In the presence of glucose, male embryos completed the first three cleavages before female embryos, but in the absence of glucose the opposite occurred. These authors also observed that the high concentration of glucose, if present only in the first twenty-four hours of development, is enough to alter the sex ratio of morulas and blastocysts on the seventh day of culture. It is known that glucose stimulates the formation of ROS (BREDBACKA & BREDBACKA, 1996 a ; b; IWATA *et al,* 1999), which in female embryos are at lower levels (PEIPPO & BREDBACKA, 1995; BREDBACKA & BREDBACKA, 1996 a ; b), and it has therefore been suggested that the difference in embryo development speed is related to this fact (BREDBACKA & BREDBACKA, 1996 a ; b).

In the experiments by Bredbacka & Bredbacka (1996 a; b) and Rheingantz *et al.* (2004), the concentration of glucose in the culture medium (5.56 mM) and oxygen in the atmosphere (20%) were the same. Rheingantz *et al.* (2004) noticed a gradual increase in the percentage of males as the embryo developed, even in the absence of glucose in the culture medium, indicating that glucose is not the only factor involved in this process.

process. Bredbacka & Bredbacka (1996 a ; b) attribute the faster development of male embryos solely to the presence of exogenous glucose in the culture medium, due to the possible role of glucose-6-phosphate dehydrogenase (G6PD). It is important to explain that G6PD is a critical enzyme that helps to detoxify reactive free radicals and lipid hydroperoxides and is more active in female embryos due to the X chromosome. This has been suggested by the fact that the average proportion of glucose metabolized via the PPP pathway is higher in female embryos than in male embryos (PEIPPO *et al.*, 2001).

1.13.3 Free radicals

Although free radicals have a cytotoxic action, they also have a stimulating effect on embryo development (RIEGER, 1992), and are found at lower levels in female embryos than in male embryos (PEIPPO & BREDBACKA, 1995; BREDBACKA & BREDBACKA, 1996 a; b).

According to Iwata *et al.* (1998), almost all cells grown *in vitro* are subject to damage from exposure to ROS, which in these systems are generated by increased oxygen pressure, reactions between cellular proteins, lipids and DNA, resulting in enzyme inactivation, lipid membrane peroxidation and DNA alterations.

Mitochondria play a fundamental role in providing energy for the embryo and may interfere with the difference in development between male and female embryos, since the greater cell proliferation in male embryos requires higher levels of cellular energy. The fact that male embryos have more copies of mtDNA indicates that mitochondrial degradation is greater in males than in females during early development, which suggests a difference in the number and/or activity of mitochondria in developing mammals of different sexes (MITTWICH, 2004).

Peippo *et al.* (2001) discuss the possibility that differences in growth rates are due to factors related to the inactivation of the X chromosome, causing different gene expressions and influencing the performance of enzymes that control reactive oxygen species (ROS). According to Rheingantz *et al.* (2004), in their experiment mentioned above, the presence of oxygen radicals in the culture medium seems to play a role in the mechanism that determines sexual deviation, which is related to the speed of development.

The high concentration of glucose can increase ROS through the xanthine oxidase - hypoxanthine reaction (XOD HXT), which is one of the major sources of ROS *in vitro* (IWATA *et al.*, 1999). As enzymes related to glucose control are over-expressed in female embryos before the inactivation of one of the X chromosomes, free radicals are found at lower levels in this genus (BREDBACKA & BREDBACKA, 1996 a ; b, PEIPPO & BREDBACKA, 1995), the enzymes are G6PDH, already mentioned and HPRT, which plays a role in the metabolization of hypoxanthine (KOCCHAR, *et al.,* 2001). The increased activity of these enzymes can delay the development of female embryos (BREDBACKA & BREDBACKA, 1996 a ; b), because, as previously mentioned, free radicals are stimulants up to a certain level (RIEGER, 1992).

More recently, Bermejo *et al.* (2008) also agreed on this issue and stated that the enzymes G6PDH and HPRT are important components of energy metabolism and are related to the control of free radicals. They also showed that these enzymes are found at higher levels in female bovine embryos.

The oxygen tension in the gas atmosphere also seems to influence the sex ratio of the embryos produced *in vitro.* It is known that a high oxygen tension in the gas atmosphere (20%) increases the generation of oxygen radicals derived from XOD-HXT reactions (IWATA *et al.*, 1999). In the experiments by Rheingantz (2004), Peippo & Bredbacka (1996) and Bredbacka & Bredbacka (1996), high concentrations of glucose in the culture medium (5.56 mM) and oxygen in the atmosphere (20%) were used, which may have led to an increase in free oxygen radicals in the culture medium, causing oxidative stress. According to Rheingantz *et al.* (2004), this could accelerate the development of male embryos by increasing the XOD-HXT reactions, even in the absence of glucose, but in its presence it would be exacerbated. In these studies, an increase of male embryos in the culture medium was observed, while females, as previously mentioned, because they have lower levels of free radicals, were found in a lower proportion.

3.3.5 Genetics

With fertilization, sexual differentiation begins in cattle, as in other mammals, so that the female embryo will have two X chromosomes while the male embryo will have one X chromosome and one Y chromosome (RUFINO, 2006). The influence of gene expression in relation to sex and its responsibility for the difference in the sex ratio of bovine embryos has been discussed.

According to Gutierrez-Adan *et al.* (2006), evidence suggests that the epigenetic differences produced by the presence of one or two X chromosomes are the main cause of the differences between males and females in the pre-implantation period. It is known that many genes with dependent gender expression are located on the X chromosome (200 genes), however, genes of the same importance are also found on the Y chromosome. It has been suggested that sex-related gene expression affects the development of embryos soon after the embryonic genome is activated (AVERY *et al.* 1989a;1992; XU *et al.*,1992).

It can be speculated that the greater expression of vital genes, located on the X chromosome, prior to the inactivation and dose compensation that occurs in females, contributes to the differential development rates observed between males and females (KOCCHAR *et al.*, 2001). This is because male embryos produced *in vitro* grow faster than female embryos during the seventh and eighth day after fertilization (AVERY *et al.* 1989a;1992; XU *et al.*,1992).Genes linked to the Y chromosome can have an "accelerating" effect on males and the two active X chromosomes can have a "retarding" effect on females during the pre-implantation period (GUTIERREZ-ADAN *et al.*, 1997).

Genetic factors can affect the basic biochemistry of embryos in the early development of males and females, with gender being specific. There are two "male-specific" factors: the expression of genes related to the Y chromosome, limited to that gender, and recessive mutations linked to the X chromosome, so all the cells of XY embryos would suffer the consequences of a mutation of a gene related to the X chromosome, while female embryos, with two X chromosomes, would suffer only in the cells that carry the mutation of the active X chromosome. There are also two specific factors in females: the expression of genes from both X chromosomes and a defect in the initiation or maintenance of the inactivation of the

X chromosome (GUTIERREZ-ADAN *et al.*, 2006).

Gutierrez-Adan *et al.* (2006) showed that the relative mRNA abundance of three genes linked to the X chromosome are expressed at higher levels in female bovine embryos at the early blastocyst stage. These genes are related to G6PD, HPRT and the apoptosis-inhibiting protein (XIAP), which, as explained above, are involved in energy metabolism and act in the control of free oxygen radicals . The same author, in another study, suggests that the difference in sex ratio may be due to the fact that two X chromosomes in the female embryo are active up to a stage, causing imbalances in carbohydrate metabolism (GUTIERREZ-ADAN *et al.*, 2002).

Differences in growth, metabolism, genetics and epigenetic programming during the pre-implantation phases indicate that males and females may respond differently according to environmental conditions and suggest that early disturbances may have a sex-specific effect not only on the pre-implantation period, but also on post-natal development (GUTIERREZ-ADAN *et al.*, 2006).

3.3.6 Sperm selection

Kochhar *et al.* (2001) suggest that one of the factors related to the sexual disproportion of embryos produced *in vitro* is the favoring of sperm carrying the Y chromosome before fertilization and preferential support after fertilization. At the moment of fertilization, the sperm contributes the X or Y chromosome, so that the complete chromosomal development of the zygote occurs (DOMINKO AND FIRST, 1997).

Sperm carrying the X or Y chromosome show differences in their ability to fertilize oocytes, which may be due to differences in motility, viability time or in the acrosome capacitation and reaction processes (GUTIERREZ ADAN *et al.*, 1999).

According to McEvoy (1992), sperm selection methods involve characteristics of sperm carrying the XeY chromosome, including mass, motility, DNA content and surface charge.

The most commonly used methods for sperm selection are *Swin Up* and Percoli (HOSSEPIAN DE LIMA *et al*., 2000).

The *Swin Up* method is based on the tendency of motile sperm to migrate upwards to the top of the medium, while sperm with lower motility and dead remain at the bottom of the medium (PARRISH *et al*., 1988). The Percoll gradient method consists of depositing the sperm on two or more layers of Percoll, with different concentrations, inside a tube, which is then subjected to centrifugation (RHEINGANTZ *et al*., 2000), allowing the sperm to be separated from the other constituents of the semen by the density of the layers (MACHADO, 2009).

McEvoy (1992) speculated that sperm carrying the Y chromosome are faster than those carrying the X chromosome, which could favor the selection of sperm carrying the Y chromosome when selected by the *Swin Up* method. In the experiment carried out by Avery *et al.* (1992) it was found that 60% of the embryos on the seventh day of culture were male, when the sperm selection method used was *Swin Up*, which is in line with the above explanation.

Rheingantz *et al.* (2000) obtained a higher percentage of male embryos when using the *Swin Up* method than with the Percoll method, in the absence of glucose, which confirms previous observations that *Swin Up* favors the selection of sperm carrying the Y chromosome, determining the production of a higher percentage of male embryos. Other studies have found the same results (PEGORARO *et al*., 2002; AVERY *et al*., 1992; RHEINGANTZ *et al*., 2004, WOLF *et al*., 2009; PEGORARO, 1988; RHEINGANTZ *et al*., 2006).

Rheingantz *et al.* (2004) observed a deviation in the proportion of males at later stages of development, especially when the sperm are selected using the *Swin Up* method *and the* zygotes are cultured in the presence of glucose.

Subsequently, Wolf *et al.* (2009) also found that semen selected by the *Swin Up* method resulted in a greater number of male embryos when compared to the Percoli gradient method.

According to Rheingantz *et al.* (2006), the Percoll gradient method should favor the selection of sperm carrying the X chromosome, which has a higher density than those carrying the Y chromosome. Heavier sperm cross the gradient more quickly than lighter sperm, so the centrifugation time should favor sperm carrying the X chromosome. The shorter the centrifugation time, the fewer sperm carrying the Y chromosome will have crossed the 90% gradient (WOLF *et al.,* 2009).

Wolf and colleagues (2009) found that semen selected using a discontinuous gradient of 45-90% Percoll (2mL) showed no variation in the percentage of male and female embryos. On the other hand, a continuous gradient of 67.5% Percoll (2 mL) produced more female embryos (63%). Iwasaki *et al.* (1988) used four Percoll gradients for sperm selection, and there was no deviation from the sex ratio.

Still on this subject, Machado (2009) discusses the impact of the longer time that the lighter sperm, the Y sperm, remain in contact with Percoll. Alterations in the sperm cells can occur due to prolonged contact, which, when placed in IVF medium, could be hyperactivated and capacitated more quickly, consequently fertilizing the oocytes before the sperm with the X chromosome. However, with a smaller volume of Percoll, neither the sperm carrying the X chromosome nor the sperm carrying the Y chromosome would take long to cross the gradient, so they would have no advantage at the time of fertilization. However, in this experiment, the author found no change in the sex ratio when the volume of the gradient was reduced from 2mL to 400 µL. In the study where the volume of Percoll was increased (8 and 12 mL) for sperm selection, 75% of female embryos were found, demonstrating that changes in the volume of Percoll can favor lighter or heavier sperm (HOSSEPIAN DE LIMA *et al.*, 2000).

3.3.7 Oocyte maturation and fertilization time

According to Machado *et al. (2009), the* duration of co-incubation of sperm and oocyte influences the sex ratio of embryos produced *in vitro*. Gamete interaction *in vitro* can affect the fertilization process by giving one sex a developmental advantage over the other, since males begin development earlier than females. Therefore, the sex ratio would depend on the stage of maturation of the oocyte and the interaction kinetics between the sperm and the oocyte (KOCCHAR *et al.,* 2001). The sequential changes to oocyte maturation and the timing of sperm addition may be of crucial importance to the oocyte's ability to activate and support embryonic development (DOMINKO AND FIRST, 1997).

In the experiment by Dominko and First (1997), it was observed that the majority of oocytes inseminated shortly after the first polar body was extruded produced a greater number of female embryos, while oocytes inseminated eight hours after extrusion developed into male embryos. Also in this study, most of the embryos that completed their first cell cycle within 30 hours of insemination were male and had a greater number of cells than the female embryos. It has therefore been suggested that the stage of maturation of the oocyte at the time of insemination may be responsible for the preferential processing of sperm carrying the Y or X chromosome.

In the Kochhar *et al.* study (2003), the results were in line with those described above, as more male embryos were produced than females when there were 6 hours of co-incubation. However, in the group with long (9, 12 and 18 h) co-incubation, there was no significant change in the sex ratio. The authors suggested that during the first six hours of co-incubation, there is probably a selective advantage between the oocyte and the sperm carrying the Y chromosome, which is more successful in fertilizing the oocytes at this stage. It is also possible that the disadvantage is due to the loss of glycoproteins during the prolonged movement of the sperm.

It is important to note that prolonged exposure of oocytes to high concentrations of sperm has a detrimental effect on fertilization and embryo development, due to the excessive production of ROS (KOCCHAR *et al.*, 2001).

4. CONCLUSION

It's important to realize the practical aspect of the work discussed, as it could lead to better use of cattle farming, by using methods that increase the proportion of a given sex, through *in vitro* embryo production, as it is a widespread technique with prospects for even greater growth. Market needs and the competitiveness imposed by the cattle industry increasingly demand herds with greater genetic potential. IVP protocols aimed at increasing the proportion of a given sex can meet the need to choose a gender of interest for each production system and genetic improvement program, helping to maximize the sector's profitability. However, in order to optimize protocols, more studies are needed, given the divergence between authors and the complexity of the subject.

5. BIBLIOGRAPHICAL REFERENCES

ASBIA. **Artificial Insemination Report.** 2011. Available at: [http://www.asbia.org.br/novo/upload/mercado/relatorio2011.pdf]. Accessed on: March 20, 2012.

AVERY B, SCHMIDT T, Greve T. Sex determination of bovine embryos based on cleavage rates. **Acta Vet Scand**;30:147-153, 1989 A.

AVERY, B.; BACK, A.; SCHMIDT, T. Differential cleavage rates and sex determination in bovine embryos. **Theriogenology**, v. 32, p. 139-147, 1989 B.

AVERY, B.; JORGENSEN, C. B.; MADISON, V.; et al. Morphological development and sex of bovine *in vitro-fertilized* embryos. **Molecular Reproduction and Development**, v. 32, p. 265-270, 1992.

BARUSELLI, P. S.; REIS, E. L.; MARQUES M. O. Management techniques to improve reproductive efficiency in *Bos indicus* females. **Grupo de Estudo de Nutriçâo de Ruminantes** - Departamento de Melhoramento e Nutriçâo Animal - FCA - FMVZ - Unesp, Botucatu, Sâo Paulo, p.18, 2004.

BARUSELLI, P. S.; AYRES, H. ; SOUZA, A. H. ; et al . Impact of IATF on reproductive efficiency in beef cattle. **In: 2nd International Symposium on Applied Animal Reproduction**, Londrina, PR. Biotecnologia da Reproduçâo em Bovinos, v.1, p.113-132, 2006.

BEARDEN, H.J.; FUQUAY, J.W. **Applied Animal Reproduction, 4th edition, Simon and Schuster Co., New York, 1997.**

BERMEJO-ALVAREZ, P.; RIZOS, D.; RATH, D.; et al. Epigenetic differences between male and female bovine blastocysts produced *in vitro*. **Physiol Genomics**, v.32, p.264-272, 2008.

BÓ, G.A.; BARUSELLI, P.S.; MARTINEZ, M.F. Pattern and manipulation of follicular development in Bos indicus. **Animal Reproduction Science**, v.78, p.307-326, 2003.

BOLS, P. E. J.; YSEBAERT, M.T; VAN SOOM, A.; et al. Effects of needle tip bevel and aspiration procedure on the morphology and developmental capacity bovine compact cumulus oocyte complexes. **Theriogenology**, Stoneham, v.47, p.1221-1236, 1997.

BREDBACKA, K.; BREDBACKA, P. Glucose controls sex-related growth rate differences of bovine embryos produced *in vitro*. **Journal Reproduction of Fertility**, v.106, p.169-172, 1996 A.

BREDBACKA, K.; BREDBACKA, P. Sex-related cleavage rate difference in bovine embryos produced *in vitro* is controlled by glucose. **Theriogenology**, v.45, n.1, p.191, 1996 B.

DIAS, J. **Brazilian bovine embryo market.** 2012. Available at: [http://www.artigonal.com/marketing-internacional-artigos/mercado-brasileiro-de-embrioes-bovinos-fiv-5799665.html]. Accessed on: October 6th. 2012.

DOMINKO, T.; FIRST, N.L.. Relationship between the maturational state of oocytes at the time of insemination and sex ratio of subsequent early bovine embryos. **Theriogenology,** v. 47, p.1041- 1050, 1997.

FERREIRA, M. B. D.; LOPES, B. C. ; FERREIRA, J. J. . Sustainability of the milk production system with F1 animals: perspectives and research. **In: Milk production and society: a critical analysis of the milk chain in Brazil.** Belo Horizonte: FEPMVZ-editora, v. 1, p. 383-404, 2001.

GALINA, C.S.; ORIHUELA, A.; RUBIO, I. Behavioral trends affecting oestrus detection in Zebu cattle. **Animal Reproduction Science**, v.42, p.465-470, 1996.

GALLI, C.; DUCHI, R.; CROTII, G.; et al. Bovine embryo technologies. **Theriogenology**, v.59, p.599-616, 2003.

GALLI, C.; LAZZARI, G. Practical aspects of IVM/IVF in cattle. **Animal Reproduction Science**, v.42, p.371-379, 1996.

GARCIA J.M.; AVELINO K.B.; VANTINI R. State of the art of *in vitro* fertilization in cattle. **In**: *Annals of the First International Symposium on Animal Reproduction Applied: Londrina.* p 223-230, 2004.

GILARDI, S.G.T. ; SA, W.F. ; CAMARGO, L.S.A.; et al. Effect of different culture media on the development and sex ratio of bovine embryos produced in vitro. **Arquivo Brasileiro de Medicina Veterinària e Zootecnia**, v. 56, n. 5, p. 623-627, 2004.

GONCALVES, P. B. D. ; BARRETA, M.H. ; SANDRI, L.R. ; et al. In vitro production of bovine embryos: the state of the art. **Revista Brasileira de Reproduçâo Animal,** v. 31, p. 212-217, 2007.

GONCALVES, P.B.D.; FIGUEIREDO, J.R.; FREITAS, V.J.F. **Biotechniques applied to animal reproduction**. Sâo Paulo:Varela, 2008.

GRISART, B.; MASSIP, A.; COLLETTE, L.; et al. The sex ratio of bovine embryos produced in vitro in serum-free oviduct cell-conditioned medium is not altered. **Theriogenology**, v. 43, p.1097-106, 1995.

GUTIERREZ-ADAN, A.; OTER, M.; MARTINEZ-MADRID, B.; et al. Differential expression of two genes located on the X chromosome between male and female in vitro-produced bovine embryos at the blastocyst stage. **Mol Reprod Dev,** v.55, p.146-151, 2000.

GUTIÉRREZ-ADÂN, A.; BEHBOODI, E.; MURRAY, J.D.; et al. Early transcription of the SRY gene by bovine preimplantation embryos. **Molecular Reproduction and Development**, v. 48, p. 246-250, 1997.

GUTIÉRREZ-ADÂN, A.; PEREZ, G.; GRANADOS, J.; et al. Relationship between sex ratio and time of insemination according to both time of ovulation and maturational state of oocyte. **Zygote**, v. 7, p. 37-43, 1999.

GUTIERREZ-ADAN, A.; BEHBOODI, E.; ANDERSEN, G.B.; et al. Relationship between stage of development and sex of bovine IVMIVF embryos cultured in vitro versus in the sheep oviduct. **Theriogenology** v.46, p. 515-525, 1996.

GUTIÉRREZ-ADÂN, A.; LONERGAN, P.; RIZOS, D. et al. Effect of the in vitro culture system on the kinetics of blastocyst development and sex ratio of bovine embryos.**Theriogenology**, v. 55, p. 1117-1126, 2001.

GUTIERREZ-ADAN, A.; PEREZ-CRESPO, M.; FERNANDEZ-GONZALEZ, R.; et al. Developmental consequences of sexual dimorphism during pre- implantation embryonic development. **Reprod. Domest. Anim.,** v. 41, Suppl 2, p. 54-62, 2006.

HAFEZ, E. S. E.; HAFEZ, B. **Folliculogenesis, egg Maturation, and ovulation**. Philadelphia: Lippincott Williams & Wilkins, 2000. Chap.5, p.68-82.

HOLM, P.; SHUKRI, N.N.; VAJTA, G. et al. Developmental kinetics of the first cell cycles of bovine *in vitro* produced embryos in relation to their *in vitro* viability and sex.

Theriogenology,v.50, p.1285-1299, 1998.

HOSSEPIAN DE LIMA, V. F. M . Methodological advances in bovine sperm sex selection for use in genetic improvement and animal production. **Revista Brasileira de Zootecnia**, v. 36, p. 219-228, 2007.

HOSSEPIAN DE LIMA, V.F.M.; RAMALHO, M.D.T.; RODRIGUES, L.H.; et al. Separation of X- and Y-bearing bovine spermatozoa by Percoll density gradient centrifugation. **Theriogenology**, v. 53, n. 1, p. 480, 2000 (abstract).

IBGE. PPM 2010: **National cattle herd grows by 2.1% to 209.5 million head.** 2011. Available at:

[http://www.ibge.gov.br/home/presidencia/noticias/noticia_visualiza.php?id_noticia=2002&id_pagina=1 e

[http://www.ibge.gov.br/home/estatistica/economia/ppm/2010/default_pdf.shtm].

Accessed on: October 5, 2012.

IWASAKI, S.; SHIOYA, Y.; MASUDA, H.; et al. Sex ratio of early embryos fertilized in vitro with spermatozoa separated by percoll. **Theriogenology**, v.30, p. 1191-1198, 1988.

IWATA, H.; AKAMATSU, S.; MINAMI, N.; et al. Effects of antioxidants on the development of bovine IVM/IVF embryos in various concentrations of glucose. **Theriogenology.** v.50, p. 365-375, 1988.

IWATA, H.; AKAMATSU, S.; MINAMI, N.; et al. Allopurinol, an inhibitor of xanthine oxidase, improves the development of IVM/IVF bovine embryos (>4 cell) *in vitro* under certain culture conditions. **Theriogenology**, v. 51, n. 3, p. 613-622, 1999.

KING, W.A.; YADAV, B.R.; XU, K.P. et al. The sex ratios of bovine embryos produced *in vivo* and *in vitro*. **Theriogenology**,v.36, p.779-788, 1991.

KOCHHAR, H. P. S.; PEIPPO, J.; KING, W. A. Sex related embryo development.

Theriogenology, v. 55, p. 3-14, 2001.

KOCHHAR, H.S.; KOCHHAR, K.P.; BASRUR, P.K; et al. Influence of the duration of gamete interaction on cleavage, growth rate and sex distribution of in vitro produced bovine embryos. **Anim. Reprod. Science,** v.77, p.33-49, 2003.

KRUIP, T. A. M.; BONI, R.; WURTH, Y.A.; et al. Potential use of ovum pick-up for embryo production and breeding in cattle. **Theriogenology**, v.42, p.675-684, 1994.

LÙCIO, A.C. **Influence of the method of separating viable spermatozoa ("swim-up") on the efficiency of bovine sex selection by discontinuous density gradient and the impact on genetic improvement**. 2007. 88p. Master's Degree Dissertation: Faculty of Sciences

Agriculture and Veterinary Sciences. Universidade Estadual Paulista Jûlio de Mesquita Filho de Jaboticabal. Jaboticabal, 2007.

MACHADO, G. M. **Effect of different Percoll protocols on sperm quality and *in vitro* production of bovine embryos**. 2009. 67p. Master's dissertation: Faculty of Agronomy and Veterinary Medicine. University of Brasilia. Brasilia, 2009.

MC EVOY, J.D. Alteration of sex ratio. **Animal Breeding Abstracts**, v.60, n.2, p.97-111, 1992.

MERIGHE, G. K. F.; MIRANDA, M. S.; DE BEM, T. H. C.; et al . Effect of passage number and gender of nucleus donor cells on the development of cattle produced by nuclear transfer**. Revista Brasileira de Zootecnia**, v. 39, p. 2166-2173, 2010.

MIES FILHO, A. **Artificial insemination**. 3.ed. Porto Alegre: Sulina, v. 2, 645p., 1975.

MINISTRY OF AGRICULTURE, LIVESTOCK AND SUPPLY (MAPA**). Brazilian Agribusiness: An Investment Opportunity.** Available at [www.agricultura.gov.br]. Accessed on: February 27, 2012.

MITTWOCH, U. The elusive action of sex-determining genes: mitochondria to the rescue? **Theriogenology**, v.228, p. 359-365, 2004.

NEVES, J . P.; MIRANDA, K. L.; TORTORELLA, R.D. Scientific progress in reproduction in the first decade of the 21st century. **Revista Brasileira de Zootecnia**, v.39, p.414-421, 2 0 1 0 (supl.especial).

PEGORARO, L. M. C. et al. Percoll gradient versus swim-up: effect of sperm preparation method on sex ratio of in vitro-produced bovine embryos. **Theriogenology**, v. 57, n. 1, p. 751, 2002 abstract

PEGORARO, L. M. C.; THUARD, J. M.; DELALLEAU, N.; et al. Comparisons of sex ratio and cell number of IVM- IVF bovine blastocysts co-cultured with bovine oviduct epithelial cells or with vero cells. **Theriogenology** 49, 15791590, 1998.

PEIPO, J.; BREDBACKA, P. Male bovine zygotes cleave earlier than female zygotes in the presence of glucose. **Theriogenology**, v. 45, n. 1, p. 187, 1996.

PEIPO, J.; BREDBACKA, P. Sex-related growth rate differences in mouse preimplantation embryos *in vivo* and *in vitro*. **Molecular Reproduction and Development**, v. 40, p. 56-61, 1995.

PEIPPO, J.; KURKILAHTI, M.; BREDBACKA, P. Developmental kinetics of in vitro produced bovine embryos: the effect of sex, glucose and exposure to timelapse environment. **Zygote,** v.9, n.2, p.105-113, 2001.

PESQUEIRO, J.B.; BAPTISTA, H.A.; MOTTA, F.L.T.; et al. **Applications of transgenic animals** . Scientific American Brasilian, v. 56, p. 78-85, 2007.

PINEDA, N. Brazilian genetic base to be multiplied**. In: International Symposium on Applied Animal Reproduction**, 1, Londrina, 2004.

RHEINGANTZ, M. G. T. ; PEGORARO, L. M. C.; DELLAGOSTIN, O. A.; et al. Male:female ratio of bovine embryos cultured in the presence or absence of glucose after IVF with spermatozoa selected by swim-up or percoll gradient. **Brazilian Journal of Veterinary Research and Animal Science**, v. 41, n. 1, p. 32-39, 2004.

RHEINGANTZ, M. G. T.; PEGORARO, L. M. C.; DESCHAMPS, J. C.; et al. Effect of sperm preparation method on sex ratio from in vitro bovine produced embryos **In. International Congress Animal Reproduction**, Stockholm, Sweden, v. 2, p. 176, 2000.

RHEINGANTZ, M. G. T.; PEGORARO, L. M. C.; Dellagostin, O.A.; et al. The sex ratio of *in vitro* produced bovine embryos is affected by the method of sperm preparation. **Animal Reproduction**, v. 3, n.4, 2006.

RIEGER, D. Relationships between energy metabolism and development of early mammalian embryos.**Theriogenology**, v. 37, n. 1, p. 75-93, 1992.

RODRIGUES, C. F. M.; GARCIA, J. M. In vitro fertilization: commercial application. **Arquivos da Faculdade de Veterinària UFRGS**, Porto Alegre, v.28, n.1,p. 186-187, 2000.

RUFINO, F.A.; SENEDA, M.M.; ALFIERI, A.A. Sex determination of bovine embryos produced *in vitro*: a review of methods with emphasis on PCR. **Archives of Veterinary Science**, v. 11, n. 1, p. 1-7, 2006.

RUMPF, R. Methodological advances *in in vitro* embryo production. **Revista Brasileira de Zootecnia**, v. 36, special supplement, p. 229-233, 2007.

RUVUNA, F.; TAYLOR, J.F.; WALTER, J.P. et al. Bioeconomic evaluation of embryo transfer in beef production systems:III. Embryo lines production bulls. **Journal of Animal Science**, v.70, p.1091-97, 1992.

MINAS GERAIS STATE SECRETARIAT OF AGRICULTURE, LIVESTOCK AND SUPPLY. **Profile of world agribusiness**. 2011 Available at:

[http://www.agricultura.mg.gov.br/files/perfil/perfil_mundial.pdf]. Accessed on: March 3,

2012.

SENEDA, M. M.; SANTOS, G. M. G.; SILVA, K. C. F.; et al. Current situation of follicular aspiration and *in vitro* fertilization. **In: II International Symposium on Applied Animal Reproduction**, 1, 2006, Londrina. **Proceedings...** Londrina, p. 172180, 2006.

SEVERO, N.C. Influence of frozen bovine semen quality on fertility. **A Hora Veterinària**, v. 28, n.167, p.36-39, 2009.

SILVA, A. S.; SILVA, E.V.C.; NOGUEIRA, E.; et al. Evaluation of the cost/benefit of conventional and fixed-time artificial insemination of multiparous beef cattle. **Revista Brasileira de Reproduçâo Animal**, v.31, n.4, p.443-455, 2007.

THIBIER, M. The zootechnical applications of biotechnology in animal reproduction: current methods and perspectives. **Reproduction, Nutrition and Development**, v. 45, p. 235-242, 2005.

TIFFIN G.J.; RIEGER D.; BETTERIDGE K.J.; et al. Glucose and glutamine metabolism in pre-attachment cattle embryos in relation to sex and stage of development. **Journal Reproduction of Fertility**, v.93, p.125-132, 1991.

VIUFF, D. et al. Transcriptional activity in in vitro produced bovine two- and four-cell embryos. **Molecular Reproduction and Development**, v.43, p.171179, 1996.

WOLF, C. A.; BRASS, K. E. ; RUBIN, M. I. B.; et al. The effect of sperm selection by Percoll or swim up on the sex ratio of in vitro produced bovine embryos. **Animal Reproduction**, v.5, p.110-115, 2008.

XU, K. P.; YADAV, B. R.; KING, W. A.; BETTERIDGE, K. J. Sex-related differences in developmental rates of bovine embryos produced and cultured *in vitro*. **Molecular Reproduction and Development**, v.31, p.249-252, 1992.

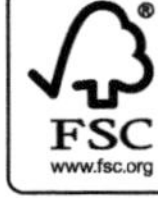

MIX
Papier aus verantwortungsvollen Quellen
Paper from responsible sources
FSC® C105338

Printed by Books on Demand GmbH, Norderstedt / Germany